A Cocoon with a View

'Remarkable.'
RTÉ.ie

'Full of charm, wit and wisdom ... As you would expect from [Alice],
it is heart-warming, inspiring and comforting.'
Irish Independent

'Fuelled by good humour and home-spun wisdom.'
Evening Echo

About Alice Taylor's other books

And Life Lights Up
'Alice's beautiful and captivating writing is an act of mindfulness in itself,
and she shares her favourite moments in life, encouraging us to ponder
our own. Alice also inspires the reader to be attentive to the here and now
and embrace moments as they arise. A beautiful and enchanting book by a
bestselling and celebrated author.'
Mummypages

Do You Remember?
'Magical ... Reading the book, I felt a faint ache in my heart ... I find
myself longing for those days ... Alice Taylor has given us a handbook for
survival. In fact, it is essential reading.'
Irish Independent

For more books by Alice Taylor, see www.obrien.ie

A Cocoon with a View

Alice Taylor

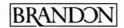

First published 2020 by Brandon,
an imprint of The O'Brien Press,
12 Terenure Road East, Rathgar,
Dublin 6, DO6 HD27, Ireland.
Tel: +353 1 4923333; Fax: +353 1 4922777
E-mail: books@obrien.ie
Website: www.obrien.ie
Reprinted 2020 (three times).
The O'Brien Press is a member of Publishing Ireland.

ISBN 978-1-78849-222-5

10 9 8 7 6 5 4
23 22 21 20

Printed and bound in Ireland by Sprint Print.
The paper in this book is produced using pulp from
managed forests.

Published in:

DUBLIN
UNESCO
City of Literature

Dedication

For Mike, and unseen family,
friends and neighbours who beam
rays of light and comfort
into my cocoon

Contents

The Invisible Visitor

Back in the last weeks of February, which now feels like a hundred years ago, we here in Innishannon were busy planning what was termed 'The Big Rake Off' of the dead grass on the long, sloping bank beside the road coming into the village. It was to be our first step in the creation of a long wildflower meadow, or bank in this case. The main aim was to sustain our bird and bee life on this curving, sloping hillside where, to mark the Millennium, we had planted many trees, and beneath them had continued to cut the grass on a regular basis. But now we were changing that approach. The new plan was the creation of a long, winding curve of beautiful wildflowers waving in the breeze – and brighten up the lives of the thousands of drivers daily whizzing by into and out of West Cork. We planned a large gathering of workers on a sunny

Saturday morning to get the wheels of this plan in motion. This long bank enjoys a south-facing, sunny location, so was the ideal place for a parish picnic that was planned as part of The Big Rake Off. The event brings to mind the lines of Thomas Gray:

Alas, regardless of their doom,
The little victims play!
No sense have they of ills to come,
Nor care beyond to-day.

Happily unaware of forthcoming events, we were totally focused on creating our wildflower bank. To get something like this going you need a '*meitheal*', a word which prior to arrival of the coronavirus was a foreign language to anyone under forty. When I used it, my daughter would tell me, 'Nobody in today's world knows the meaning of that word.' Amazing that the coronavirus has resurrected it simply because we are now one great *meitheal*, united in fighting this invisible enemy.

But before this virus turned ordinary life on its head, we were in the process of rounding up a *meitheal*. To round up a *meitheal* you need to alert all potential helpers that their presence is required on a specified date. In our village, the first step in achieving this is the Village Pole, which very obligingly stands on a corner right in the centre of the village. On it, all clubs pin their posters of future plans and hope that passersby will get the message. The second channel of communication is the church *Newsletter*, from which the church-goers will hopefully spread the word. Then on to the local press, which for us is the *Southern Star* and the *Examiner*. We seldom make the main *Examiner* itself, unless we have done something to upset the nation or said something newsworthy. But we are extremely grateful to get into their weekly supplement, *The County*.

Have patience with me now as I will eventually get to the point! I regularly need to say the prayer: 'Lord, give speed to my tongue to get straight to the point!' But, sure, now we have lots of time because no one is in a hurry. That is the biggest thing about living in cocooning territory – there is no hurry.

To get into *The County*, Ailín Quinlan is our conduit and she invariably comes to our rescue. So, after a long conversation with Ailín about The Big Rake Off, the chat turned to other things, which led to a discussion of another nature, and to fill you in on the source of this discussion I need to take you back to the previous Sunday – a small bit of meandering, but I'm getting there, I promise!

That day on my way to the wood I walked through the village carpark, which, due to the recent opening of our new playground, has drawn a lot of outsiders into the village. Because we are a small village accustomed to saluting each other, the newcomers are also acknowledged. This is the way with rural living!

However, on this particular day my sometimes absent brain was switched on and I began to observe some blank faces wearing masks of non-acknowledgement pass me by. Well, I thought, what is all this about? Is this new or has it crept in stealthily without my being aware of it? A dog trotting behind one stony-faced couple wagged his tail at me – I was glad that at least the dogs had not lost their friendliness! Thinking about this new shift in our culture, I walked over the bridge across the river Bandon on my way to nearby Dromkeen Wood. As you walk over this bridge there is a lovely view, both up-river to Bandon and down-river to Kinsale, so I leant over the bridge to watch the water and soak up the view. Down below on the river bank was a pretty blond girl accompanied by a beautiful blond dog. They were both elegantly turned out in almost colour-coordinated outfits. Very impressive! The dog was having great fun jumping in and out of the water, but the pretty owner was so immersed in her mobile phone that she was totally oblivious to the dog and to her wonderful woodland surroundings. I waved down and received a puzzled frown in return. The dog wagged his tail and barked.

Finally I got to the wood. In there the atmosphere was completely different. People were smiling and friendly, the children and dogs running around and obviously having a great time. Was it the wood that was having this effect? Or do a different kind of people visit woods, I wondered? I simply don't know!

So I told Ailín about my experience and we discussed the situation, wondering if we Irish were losing our sense of connectedness and friendliness. Was it simply slipping away without us even noticing? She too had noticed the change and so she rang the main paper and asked if they would be interested on a feature about the matter. And they were! The editor felt that a lot of people were noticing what we were talking about.

So Ailín wrote her piece and on Wednesday I was the page-three girl, but with all my clothes on; perish the thought of the alternative! I was not aware that the article had appeared that morning, but on my way to Mass a friend greeted me with a big grin on her face: 'Ryan Tubridy was talking about you this morning.'

'Oh my God! What was he saying?' I asked in alarm. 'That we're not saluting each other in Innishannon!' she laughed.

But the feature rang a bell with a lot of people and many radio stations countrywide called me to discuss the matter, and it became apparent that from all around the country people were noticing our fading friendliness. Sometime later the *Today Show* from RTE TV made contact and it was arranged that I would go into their station in Cork to discuss the matter with Maura and Daithi.

In the meantime the coronavirus was stealthily advancing in our direction and on Thursday, 12 March 2020, before I left home, the researcher Nessa McLoughlin rang to ask if I was okay to travel. That made me aware that we were sailing into uncharted waters.

The discussion with Maura and Daithi that was supposed to be about our fading friendliness focused instead on the incoming treacherous tide that was steadily creeping in our direction. I came home on the evening of 12 March and after coming in my side door, which is the one we all use, I locked it! Locking that door was a strange feeling because when I am at home I never lock it. To me living behind a locked door would feel a bit like being in jail. And who would want to live like that? What kind of a life would that be? I was about to find out. An invisible enemy stalking the country had to be locked out. For the first time ever I was about to find out what life was like behind closed doors.

Home Alone

Am I cocooning or self-isolating? In today's climate both words mean the same thing, but it's amazing the different picture each word paints in our subconscious. Isolation brings to mind punishment by solitary confinement, whereas cocooning paints a picture of self-caring and nurturing. Cocooning comes from the natural world of butterflies and beehives, and the dictionary defines it as to 'envelop in a protective and comforting way'. Wouldn't that terminology make anyone feel better! So, maybe we who are advised to do so, may choose to think of cocooning instead of isolating. Perception is everything! In the brood chamber of the beehive the baby bees are cocooned until they are able to fly and fend for themselves. The caterpillars self-cocoon until they are ready to fly high as butterflies. But the difference between us and the baby bees and butterflies is that cocooning is their natural habitat, preparing them for progression into the wider world, whereas we who were flying high now have to go into reverse and fly backwards. Can we butterflies be transformed into contented caterpillars? Possibly not an easy process as we may be about to find out in the days ahead. But for the moment it's 'One Day at a Time.'

Those of us who are not cocooning are caring and sharing – from a distance. You may recall the popular song 'From a Distance', which people can now sing with a pleasant smile if and when someone is not maintaining the advised distance. The beautiful words of this song are both disturbing and prophetic, describing the beauty and bounty of a natural, peaceful world where we love and cherish each other and God is watching us from a distance. It tells of peace, hope and brotherhood, where all live in harmony. But then we blew it and the writer wonders why. That song is really an anti-war song, but it mentions marching together in a common band. Never was this more needed!

We have been parachuted into a scary new place and we are all endeavouring not to be overwhelmed. But if we over-think things, that is exactly what will happen. Our thoughts could so easily overwhelm us. The coronavirus may attack our bodies, but if we let it invade our minds too it could destroy our sense of wellbeing, which could well make us paranoid. So we are involved in two battles: the physical and the mental.

Now is a very good time to be living on a farm, as out there is the calmness and healing of nature and the animal world. A few years ago a young farmer who was on the grief road after the death of his wonderful wife told me that the animals helped him to endure and survive those brutal first days, weeks and months of bereavement. Animals and nature can stoically absorb our tumultuous emotions and erratic upheavals, and help to centre and calm us.

One morning recently on RTE radio's 'Sunday Miscellany' there was a beautifully written and very wise item by a man about doing mindfulness with four donkeys. I laughed out loud listening to it. The story-teller, because that is what he was, had read Jon Kabat-Zinn, the top guru on mindfulness, so he knew what he was talking about. He told about standing with his four donkeys in a shed on a wet day looking out to sea, and how the absolute solidity and mindfulness of the donkeys was total. It was one of the most hilarious and riveting moments that I had ever listened to on radio. It made for mesmerising listening and was full of deep wisdom. Radio moments like that are golden, especially when you are cocooning.

But we are not all lucky enough to be on farms, or to have donkeys, so it is good to have a garden or to be within the prescribed access distance to a wood, river, seaside or quiet by-road, and many roads are now a lot quieter and safer for walking.

Some years ago we had a retired hospital matron working with us helping run our guest house, and whenever a crisis occurred she would simply stand back and calmly say, 'Now, what's to be done?' And a plan of action came into play. She was accustomed to handling emergencies.

So, in the present circumstances it's a case of 'What's to be done?' And undoubtedly the first thing to be done is to do exactly as we are being told. Our government and health services are doing an amazing job, and the best and only thing for each one of us to do is exactly as they are instructing, which is changing from day to day. They have our best interests at heart and want us to survive to tell the tale.

Having ascertained the correct amount of necessary information, I feel that an overload of unnecessary news could damage our sense of wellbeing. So, maybe better not to immerse ourselves in a constant flow of coronavirus news. Best to keep ourselves occupied, doing selected projects, as there is therapy in doing.

A Cocoon with a View

I was listening to Patricia Scanlan talking to Miriam O'Callaghan on radio one Sunday morning, and she suggested making your bed each morning in the cocoon before leaving your bedroom. She was passing on a bit of helpful advice that had been given to her. It was a Sunday morning so I was relaxing in bed listening to the radio. But when I got out of bed I made it immediately and have done so every morning since. Thank you, Patricia, and Miriam! A very small thing in the bigger scheme of things, but we are living at a time when little things mean a lot. It is the little things that will keep us all sane and able to cope.

And people are doing amazing things. Every day we hear of kindness and goodness coming to the fore. How great is that! Families and friends are reaching out to each other and supporting each other. We can really be wonderful when we take the time, time to talk to each other on the phone, time to email each other and even taking the time to sit down and write letters. In these stressful times how lovely it is to get a letter.

There was a time when it was not uncommon to hear someone singing or whistling as they worked or even when out walking. We seem to have lost that one! It was a very cheery sound and wouldn't it be lovely to hear it again? It would cheer us all up, both the singer and the listener – cheer us up and lighten our hearts. In Italy during lockdown they used their balconies to sing and comfort each other. The Italians may be better singers than we are, but we have plenty of good singers too – and even songs from the few crows amongst us would not go amiss right now. Or if you have an upstairs window, why not call down and salute the passersby, and if you are a passerby why not wave and call back up. Not normal behaviour, but these are not normal times. But even in normal times we all need friendship and connectedness, though so much more so now.

There are so many things that we plan to do 'someday when we have the time'. Well, maybe the time is now. Kindness and generosity of spirit take thought and time, and now we have plenty of both. Maybe now is the time if there is a family rift or old grudge between people to let it dissolve and evaporate. How trivial are old sores in this new order.

Many years ago in Lough Derg I picked up a leaflet that I afterwards lost, but still remember the words:

We have careful words for the strangers,
And smiles for the sometime guest

A Cocoon with a View

But for our own the bitter tone
Though we love our own the best.

Ah! lips with curve impatient
Eyes with that look of scorn,
'Twere a cruel fate were the night too late
To undo the work of the morn.

How many go forth in the morning
Who never come home at night,
And hearts have broken for harsh words spoken
That sorrows can never put right.

On RTE TV recently there was a programme in which a woman told a story about a neighbouring couple who had not talked to each other directly for years. They addressed each other through the dog! And when the dog died they were in big trouble! Sounds hilarious, but how many families have had big fallouts over the years, and now children are not talking to parents or siblings to each other? Is now the time to make a move? Maybe best not to wait until the dog dies.

Matters that were convulsing the world just a few weeks ago are now totally eradicated from our consciousness. This new reality has focused us all in one direction: survival is the name of the game, and nothing focuses the mind like our own mortality.

But what a blessing that it is not the young who are in the greatest danger and also that we are facing into the summer months. The good light of summer will lift our spirits when we can go out into the great outdoors. And while out there let's not block our ears and eyes to its healing, soothing, calming essence. Be there!

Cocooning and caring and sharing at a safe distance is the new order. By all singing from the same hymn sheet, following government guidelines and helping our wonderful health-care workers by caring for ourselves and those who need us, we will one day look back and be proud of how great we were during this crisis.

Panic Buying

For some reason beyond all understanding the panic buying of toilet rolls accompanies the early days of the corona virus. There is no rational explanation for this as diarrhoea is not one of the side effects of corona, but this panic buying of toilet rolls brings back echoes of the bread-buying frenzy that was part of the Big Snow experience a while ago. Some things are beyond all explanation or understanding. Though I doubt that this was what St Paul had in mind when he told us 'understand it even though it is beyond all understanding ... '

Now, I have to admit that I did my own share of panic buying. But for me it wasn't toilet rolls but packets of sweet-pea seeds that were the object of my 'have to have' panic buying. You might well wonder why sweet peas. Have I nothing else to be worried about? But an explanation is forthcoming!

I must be one of the most well-placed cocooners

in the county! My home is on the corner of the village with three large south-facing windows onto a busy street and the main road into West Cork, which scene is now changing daily. Over the stone wall of the pub yard across the road is a great view of Dromkeen Wood, which is now putting on its summer wear, and if I go upstairs that view gets even better. At the top of my stairs is an art room converted from two surplus bedrooms where I pretend to be an artist. I am not an artist but a putter of paint on canvas, and I hope for miracles to happen – and sometimes they do, but very rarely. More often than not it's a case of blood, sweat and tears! And disasters! Nevertheless, up there I have moments of pure exultation and when inspiration fails I can look across at the wood and sometimes catch glimpses of the swans rising awkwardly out of the Bandon river and winging their way up-stream. In flight they are a majestic sight.

Stuck on top the easel at the moment is a beautiful photograph of a hare poised for flight, which I am hoping to transfer onto canvas. He has been perched up there for a long time, but one day, when the mind moves in that direction, we will take off. In the meantime, any time I pop into the room he fills me with anticipation because he and I are slowly getting to know each other. When the time comes for take-off we will be dancing in harmony because he will have taken up residence and built a home in my head and hopefully will ease his way out onto the canvas. Also up there, in waiting, is a card showing a flock of geese in full flight, but these will be a harder nut to crack. In real life geese are totally contrary, but I was reared with them and have had a long-lived love affair with them. This card, which I got from my sister who understands my nostalgic love for them, will be incredibly difficult to convey to canvas because of the varying shades of white and cream – still, they are a joy to behold, and in the meantime the anticipation of painting them is wonderful.

Anticipation

The joy of anticipation
Awaiting dreams' realisation,
Looking forward is the fun
Of happy things yet to come.

My bedroom is at the back of the house and just beside it is a glass door leading onto a flat roof where a rooftop garden has been created – that is a rather grand name for a collection of old boxes and pots, and a trellised wall which is the climbing assister for my sweet peas. Here in this warm, sunny corner, the sweet peas climb throughout the summer and fill the air with their delicious fragrance, and when snipped and brought inside they give a repeat performance in the bedroom. Then, the more you cut sweet peas the more they flower! You cannot get a performer better than that. A summer without sweet peas is to me a drab prospect, but a cocooning summer without them would be unbearable.

Down in the back yard are two large recycled plastic tubs brought to me by Paddy after his cows had demolished their contents. Paddy has access to the local Coop so I send him an SOS for potting compost and a generous supply of sweet-pea seeds. Farmers think big, so many bags of compost and an ample supply of sweet peas duly arrive: climbing sweet peas, hanging-basket peas and everlasting sweet peas. In other words, all kinds of sweet peas. I feel reinforced to cocoon with colour and fragrance.

For March the weather is unbelievably beautiful and so every morning I am out with my bucket, trowel and basket of sweet-pea packets. First port of call are the cow tubs, and having filled the base from my own compost heap I top up with the fresh potting compost, and then comes the usual search for climbing supports for the pyramids. Last year's pyramid became a bit wonky when overpowered with abundant sweet peas, so there is need for stronger thinking this year. A search of the garden shed ensues and to my delight leads to the unearthing of a large number of retired brush handles that over the years have lost their heads. Sometimes being a hoarder might be considered undesirable, but not at a time of cocooning, because now things previously seen as useless become invaluable. So, out come the handles and the makings of two stalwart pyramids, capable of bearing the most massive burden, is completed. In around them go the sweet pea seeds that I hope will climb and flower to brighten up the cocooning days ahead, however long that may be! But best not to think about that ... On the home farm long ago we had a helper, Dan, who when we children were confronted with the tough task of picking spuds or thinning turnips starting from the bottom of a long field that seemed to stretch ahead of us forever, advised: 'Head down, arse to the wind and keep going.' Dan's advice surely applies now.

Other suitable sweet-pea containers, including old tubs and battered buckets, are brought to the fore and when I run out of brush handles I fall back on bamboos and the old reliables – trunks of former Christmas trees – some of which are now looking pretty decrepit. When all are planted up, I stand back and glow with the anticipation of a yard full of masses of magnificent sweet peas. But, of course, there are hazards to be overcome, like late frost, thirst and slugs, but, fortunately enough, the dreaded weevil and red spider have no appetite for sweet peas.

Then suddenly I notice that the old table beside the shed is ominously sagging in the middle. Sitting on top of this are three heavy planters full of sweet-pea seeds that will eventually climb up the side of the shed. In the fever of planting I had failed to observe the treacherous table sag. Images of a sudden collapse when all the sweet peas are in full flower arrest me in my tracks. I poke around in the shed again and breathe a sigh of relief when I unearth two big old boxes swathed in cobwebs. I brace myself to lift the three heavy planters of sweet peas off the table, which tests my muscles almost beyond their capabilities, but eventually the planters hit the ground with a thump. I brute-force the boxes in under the table top, hoping that it will not crack up in the process, and eventually, to my relief, a level, firm table is achieved and back up go the planters of sweet peas with much huffing and puffing. Nightly on TV, fitness experts are advising us about keeping mobile while cocooning. Fitness is built into gardening, though it might kill you in the process!

Then for the low-growing sweet peas, and they go into the hanging baskets around the yard. Last year I discovered by sheer accident that they did a great job in the hanging baskets. And finally the everlasting sweet peas. Now, I am not mad about those because I have found they are all greenery with few flowers, but despite this in they go to a redundant tub because beggars can't be choosers and neither can cocooners.

Days Like This!

As soon as I open my eyes I sense a change. My inner glow has faded and cabin fever is trying to break into my cocoon. Two weeks into cocooning and this is the first morning that this has happened. My mind is a light shade of grey – and going greyer by the minute, and the challenge is to stop the surge. Cocooning is beginning to feel like isolation.

I am missing everyone! Mostly my grandchildren, seven-year-old Ellie and three-year-old Tim, who live up the hill and whom I have not hugged for two weeks. They come to the window to wave and Ellie dances with delight to entertain me, but little Tim stares in at me with a slightly confused look on his face and you can see that he is thinking: 'What is all this about?' One wonders what memory he will have of his cocooning Nana. I had taken their energising and vibrant physical presence and stimulation so much for granted. Now that it is gone I realise how life-enhancing it has been.

But the one I miss most of all is the baby, little Conor, who was born on the last day of the 2019. Because they live just up the hill I was a constant caller and he was a regular visitor to my house. A new baby is such a comfort and joy! The smell of them and the soft feel of them. The power of soft as the ad says. But now I no longer feel the power of soft. I view him on the laptop and he is growing bigger before my eyes. He and I will never have this time back.

But I cannot go down that avenue of thought. I need 'to get off that bus' and stop thinking about what is missing in my life. Must change the palette before it goes darker.

I reach my hand out and press the button on the old laptop, which is now a CD player on the bedside table, and switch on my CD on mindfulness that has so often before kicked the day into a good start. But not this morning – and after a few minutes I realise that it is just not going to happen today. Why? Because parked inside in my head is a sergeant major directing traffic – the wrong way! And, boys oh boys, is he issuing orders! And he won't stop! So I pick up my journal and pour my head into it.

That is the beauty of a journal. You can complain, rave and rant and upset no one in the process and you definitely feel better once you get all that is bothering you out of your mind. The journal absorbs your inner upheaval. It works! But don't take my word for it. Try it. Penning your thoughts onto the page succeeds in hooking that slippery grey slimy eel of unease that is slithering around in your mind, and writing it down manoeuvres it out of your head. You get better at that kind of fishing with practice. Once the lump of unease is hooked out and landed between the pages of the journal, my head is better.

This done, I kick myself out of bed, look out the window and suddenly realise that outside the sun is shining and it is a gorgeous day. Wow! But sitting on the side of the bed I suddenly notice unusual small marks on the sheet and think: What the hell is that? The experts had said nothing about bleeding to death with the coronavirus!

Then suddenly remember that last night I had put aloe vera on the backs of my hands because they were scratched from pruning roses without garden gloves – how stupid was that? Before going into bed I had reached up to the aloe vera plant on top of the chest of drawers and snipped a bit off it and applied it to the backs of my hands. During the night it must have got on to the sheet. I feel so relieved to have pinned down the reason for the dodgy-looking sheets. For a while there I thought that my days were numbered! Corona could make you paranoid!

Then comes a sudden surge of enthusiasm and I whip the sheets and pillowcases off the bed, throw them in a heap on the floor and then open all the windows onto the back garden, and drape the pillows and duvet out the windows. Already I am beginning to feel better!

Straight downstairs and into the washing machine with the sheets, pillow cases, towels, and other bits and pieces. During normal times, but mostly in winter, my washing is dried on a rack over the sink in a store room off the kitchen. But winter is gone and these are certainly not normal times, so out into the back yard go the washed sheets, towels, pillow cases. On a sudden longing to hug nature I head for the garden and drape a sheet over a stout shrub able to bear its weight, and then look around for another solid upstanding one that could also take weight. And there it is, my old faithful Louise, who has just finished flowering, so I drape a sheet over her too and she suddenly becomes a pristine, lumpy bride. The sheets glow in the sunlight. They trigger off forgotten memories. Back on the farm when my mother's long wire clothes lines were insufficient for her needs, the hedges and bushes were brought into action. There is something uplifting about the sight of white sheets spread out on bushes where the sun will do the drying. I have always loved the sight of clothes lines of washing blowing in the breeze, even in other people's gardens. The warmth of nature dries the sheets, but the sight warms your heart in the process.

The day is getting better by the minute.

For the smaller items I have an ancient timber clothes horse acquired in a junk shop a long time ago. For years it leant against a wall in the back porch and I had often wondered what the hell had ever possessed me to buy it. But eventually its time has come. That's the thing about being a hoarder. It may take some acquisitions a long time to find their niche, but when eventually they do you feel a glow of the deepest self-righteous satisfaction.

My garden, that was once full of sunlight, is now a shaded woodland, which is lovely and restful, but limits its drying facilities. However, my drying requirements have also shrunk as I am now the only occupant of the nest. So my timber clothes horse has now come into action. This clothes horse also has the added bonus that it is light, mobile and can follow the sun. There is something deeply satisfying in the sight of clothes drying in the sun on a lovely summer's day. Maybe buried deep within me is a washer-woman seeking a place in the sun!

This day is getting even better.

Back upstairs I decide to turn my large mattress over. This rattles the stuffing out of me, whatever about the mattress. When the awkward mattress finally collapses into the desired location, so do I into my rocking chair by the window. On the floor around this chair I keep a pile of favourite books for reading on just such occasions. Time to take a break! The last thing needed now is a sudden heart attack or a brain clot from over-exertion. Death, even in normal circumstances, is highly undesirable, but in the present climate would be a complete disaster and my crew would certainly not thank me for inflicting a funeral on them right now. I, who years ago had written the following poem:

Please Cry

Don't stand dry-eyed
Around my grave.
Bathe me
In the love I gave.

Pour your tears
On the earth below
To soften the thud
As down I go.
The only funeral
I would fear:
Where ne'er a one
Would share a tear.

Fat chance of tears right now should I make a sudden and what they would certainly consider an avoidable exit. They would probably think that I should have had more sense than tearing around the house and turning over a heavy mattress like a crazy woman. Maybe I might never have a tearful funeral, but I would have a much better chance in normal circumstances. And at the moment circumstances are far from normal. So best take a breather and recover my equilibrium.

There on the floor is John O'Donohue's *Benedictus*, Sarah Ban Breathnach's *Simple Abundance* and Billy Collins's *Sailing Alone Around the Room*, as well as a battered old copy of *Into the Woods* dated 1974, the oldest friend. I do a lucky-dip reading into them all, going with whatever page opens to the touch. But that does not work with Sarah because she is a day book, with a book marker for specified days. So let's see what Sarah, who is American, has to say about Friday, 27 March when she was compiling this book back in 1996, with not a whiff of corona or Trump on the horizon. Sarah quotes from George Eliot: 'It's never too late to be what you might have been.' Wouldn't that give you food for thought? Have I any idea what I might have been? Or am I about to find that out while cocooning? Could cocooning be a voyage of self-discovery?

But whatever about my journey into self-discovery, now is not the time for it, so I get my butt out of the rocking chair lest the mood to 'keep going' might evaporate. Doing things when in the mood makes all the difference, so best keep moving while the body feels that way inclined. Tomorrow this urge may well have passed.

My eye falls on two jugs of dead flowers, so down-stairs and out the back door and under a hedge in the garden with them. There is nothing more mind-deadening than dead flowers. They are an insult to the garden that grew them. Then a quick tidy-up down-stairs, when books get put in their place as well as any-thing else that is not where it should be. When I get bogged down in writing I can develop into what my grandmother termed a 'slut'. She often told me that there was nothing got from idleness but 'dirt and long nails' and she would definitely consider putting your feet up and reading or writing a book in daylight hours a highly questionable practice. So today my long-gone grandmother is dictating the pace. Out comes the vacuum cleaner and buzzes around the house. Then I polish the furniture with beautifully smelling hand-made polish purchased the last time that I visited the Ballymaloe shop. All done, I feel fulfilled and virtuous. A case of tidy your house, tidy your mind!

While all this is going on I make occasional forays out into the yard and garden to check the drying process and to do turn-overs when required. The bed linen is absorbing the smells of the garden. It is lovely to bury your face in drying bed linen and breathe in the outdoor essence. Nothing compares to the healing power of nature, especially in a cocoon.

It is now time to go back upstairs and make my bed. I am a bed person and a lover of good bed linen. We spend so much of our time in our beds that our bed linen needs to be the best we can afford. If you live alone, as I do, your bed is probably no longer a place for 'extra-curricular' activities and so may have become a place of restful communication with your-self. A place to read, write, meditate, listen, dream and sleep. And your bedroom a haven of peace – and a cocooner needs a haven.

So in come the duvet and pillows from basking in the fresh air, now smelling fresh with the warmth of the sun and the outside world. Best fresh bed linen is sourced and the bed is dressed with loving care. Tonight I will sleep in the smell of the outdoors. How great will that be! This day has been redeemed.

Confusion in the Cocoon

My laptop is having a melt-down. That scares the living daylights out of me, so when she has a melt-down I have an accompanying one. She controls my writing life and we both know that she is the smart one and I am the dopey one. This puts me in a very vulnerable situation, something akin to a master-and-slave relationship. And she takes full advantage of her status. I always really knew that I should have gone for a proper computer training course, but instead I muddled my way through managing this monster on my own. On days like this that stupid decision is deeply regretted. This is akin to owning a Doberman who tries to dominate you, and I should know all about that. When Kate came to me she was a strong-willed, powerful animal, and a smart son warned me that if I did not let Kate know who was boss she would be the master and make my life a misery. Forewarned was forearmed, so I took Kate on, and after a few challenging encounters she backed off and accepted that acquiescence was the name of the game and that there could be only be one Mastermind in the house.

I never achieved that relationship with my Apple. Every so often she does the dog and growls at me, refusing to comply with my wishes. This is one of those times. And right now, with corona already in control, her timing is brutal. She is holding my manuscript and refuses point blank to allow me in. I am scared witless that she will go thick and delete! She growls at me and flashes a warning sign about 'alias' something or other, which is totally beyond my comprehension. This petrifies me still more into slavish submission, terrified that she will gobble up weeks of work and irretrievably swallow it. Last night she began to flex her muscles and I should have smelt trouble ahead: I could not open Mail and when I cracked that one, she ground her jaws tight and would not let Mail go. Then I had to opt for Shut Down, and Mail refused to shut, so I had to Force Quit – and that drives Apple stone mad altogether. It was like facing Kate with bared teeth before she had learned who was boss. My Apple knows that *she* is the boss, so this morning when asked to comply by allowing me in, she bares her teeth at me.

Normally, my computer-smart daughter is summoned to the rescue. But these are not normal times. I am almost as terrified of losing my manuscript as I am of corona. Though not quite! I could always do a rewrite, but with corona there might be no second chance. Not a comforting thought.

So I ring my daughter and get the answering machine. I swallow an unprintable word and leave a message! Then I ring my son-in-law, who is working from home. I seldom annoy him in case of becoming a dreaded mother-in-law. Another answering machine! I leave another message. They will probably think that the house is on fire. My problem-solving daughter lives up the hill and in normal times would be down in a jiffy. But now I am cocooning and my house is off limits to her. In fact, it is off limits to everybody except Mike, who keeps me fed and watered. My daughter will think from all these phone calls that I am having a heart attack. Then my phone rings and it is my daughter with alarm in her voice. I explain my predicament and she gives a sigh of relief and placates in a soothing voice: 'Now, Mom, your manuscript is in there somewhere and it is only a matter of finding it.' I am not convinced! My daughter is of the computer generation and I am fresh off Noah's Ark. She regards the Apple as a simple machine of which she is in total command. Even seven-year-old Ellie has a similar approach. But to me my Apple is a conniving megalomaniac intent on getting the better of me.

Lena issues a few complicated instructions – at least complicated to my non computer-compliant brain – and then she realises that this is not going to work. Her mother is not getting it! So she goes on to a plan B: 'Open the side door. Put your laptop on the washing machine in the store room and you stay below in the kitchen well away from me. I will come down, sanitise my hands and sort out the problem, and then sanitise the laptop and leave.' I breathe a sigh of relief.

I put the offending laptop on the washing machine and gingerly turn the key in the side door and nervously have a peep outside, half-expecting to see Tony Holohon, Simon Harris and Leo Varadkar wagging disapproving fingers at me.

Lena arrives fitted out as if for major surgery and in a few minutes slaps my brazen Apple into submission. I remain at a distance, but it is so good to see her. Seeing her on screen and through the window is good, but this is better. Once she has gone, I lock the door.

One wonders if when corona is finally evicted,

whenever that may be, will we cocooners be like the calves and chickens in summer when the doors of their houses are opened for the first time – they stand there transfixed by the light of the great outdoors and wonder is it safe to venture out. Will we be like them?

Delighted to be united with my manuscript, but shocked by the possibility of losing it, I decide that it is time for a comforting cup of tea and so prepare a tray and take it outside. Normally I am an up-the-garden diner, but for some reason after this shockingly narrow escape with electronic erosion I need cosseting, so I opt for a cosy corner of the yard by the garden shed, just behind the back door.

The sun is warm on my face and the birds are singing. Soon I become aware as I sit there that all around me, moving from plant to plant and investigating the budding leaves, are many bees. I'm delighted to see them. Just outside the village are a few beekeepers, and bees can travel three miles from their hive for nectar. I am so glad that they have come to my garden. It gives an added satisfaction to gardening to know that you are providing food for them. All around me the red and yellow tulips are glowing in the sun, the red in full costume and the more meek yellows making a gentler statement. The reds are the front-row chorus girls, whereas the more demure yellows stand back a little from their flamboyant sisters. With autumn planting of tulips you reap a rich spring reward, and how much more appreciated is that reward this year. Little did I realise when doing the autumn planting how much they would enrich these days of cocooning. The beautiful colours sustain my spirit.

Just then I spot a new little visitor with a red hat. First saw him a few day ago – just as I came out the back door he flitted from the Olearia tree in the yard onto the roof. I had never before seen a bird like this. Or could it be that he had come other summers but because life was so busy his presence had passed unnoticed? True for Thomas Gray:

Full many a gem of purest ray serene
The dark unfathomed caves of ocean bear
How many a flower is born to blush unseen
And waste its sweetness in the desert air.

Or, as my more prosaic grandmother might put it, 'casting pearls before swine.' Now through the tree branches I see his little red hat bobbing about and hold my breath in case I frighten him. And then, to my delight, I see another. So, there is a pair. Could they be nest site-hunting? When they fly off, I take a bird feeder off the wall of the back porch and hang it on an inner branch of the tree – just to let the red-hatted pair know that a site is available with free meals attached, and that they are welcome to build here and avail of all the facilities. I will have to wait and see.

Let's Light a Candle

Every autumn flower boxes go out onto my front window-sills to brighten up the street corner and also to colour my view from inside. We need this much more during the cold grey days of winter than in summer when nature herself does it for us. Window boxes planted in the autumn pay rich dividends in both winter and spring. Each year they are a gift, but this year, blighted by corona, they are truly manna in the desert. During this winter these boxes sprouted primulas and in the bleak period from January to March, daffodils and tulips pushed up their cheery heads, urging us to hang in there.

When my window boxes were planted there was not a glimmer of corona on the horizon but during the early days of her arrival it was comforting to look out the window and see the bright primulas and stalwart golden daffodils glowing outside. Then came the elegant tulips, who were the final chorus of the flowering parade.

But with the approach of Easter the gallant tulips began to lose their elegance and flop all over the place like wavering drunks. The window boxes' days were done and they were no longer brightening up their surroundings. The last thing needed in the present climate are sad, dehydrated window boxes. So, time to bring them in! Easier said than done when cocooning. That is why the decision is fermenting in my brain for a few days before I finally get around to putting it into action.

Then early one morning before heading downstairs I do the rounds of the windows and lift in all the upstairs boxes. I line them up in a back bedroom to be dealt with *lá eile*. But bringing in the downstairs boxes and hanging baskets is a more complicated procedure. I look out at my window boxes like a cow behind an electric fence. Going out into the street is one of the many freedoms that I had so taken for granted! But now a new plan is required. So I ring grandson Fionn, who lives around the corner, with the instruction to collect all the window boxes plus hanging baskets and plonk them inside my yard gate. And then to brush down the window sills. I restrain the urge to request a wash-down of the sills, judging that to be a step too far. My grandmother had always advised cutting your cloth according to your measure!

It is the eve of Palm Sunday with Easter on the horizon, and an acknowledgement of the time that's in it is in the air. I am not a great Easter person and for me it is a time of mixed emotions, which brings to mind Chesterton's poem:

The Donkey

When fishes flew and forests walked
And figs grew upon thorn,
Some moment when the moon was blood
Then surely I was born.

With monstrous head and sickening cry
And ears like errant wings,
The devil's walking parody
On all four-footed things.

The tattered outlaw of the earth,
Of ancient crooked will;
Starve, scourge, deride me: I am dumb,

I keep my secret still.

Fools! For I also had my hour;
One far fierce hour and sweet:
There was a shout about my ears
And palms before my feet.

Always feel that this poem, full of compressed emotions, captures the turbulence of the Easter period.
That our Easter Rising in 1916 took place at this time
of year is symbolic, for me. Easter was a time of turmoil
– of death and resurrection – as indeed was the Easter
Rising, and now this current Easter the world is in the
turmoil of corona. Back in 1916 Yeats penned 'a terrible beauty is born' and one feels that at this moment
too something terrible is happening in the world. Are
we going through a crucifixion and will there be a
resurrection? A resurrection of a new respect for the
earth and its people? Right now, during these terrible
times, great kindness for the vulnerable is unfolding.

Kindness

The goodness of your kindness
Kept me in my mind,

A Cocoon with a View

Its worth could not be measured
It had goodness undefined.
You held out a caring hand
When I was full of pain,
You thawed my frozen being
And made me live again.

I wrote that when a dear friend died. At his funeral, his brother, who was a priest, gave a beautiful eulogy. He spoke of the kindness of the landscape where they had both spent their childhood. His statement warmed the heart of many in the congregation who knew that particular landscape, but had never before heard it so described. It was an apt description of a place that was kind to nature, man and beast.

Could we, perhaps, come out of this pandemic with a new sense of kindness and respect for each other and for the earth? A line from a prayer that my mother used to say comes back to me: 'And you shall renew the face of the earth.' Is the face of the earth being healed and renewed while our world stands still in the grip of corona?

When we were young and trouble came, my mother would light a candle. The first time I remember this happening was when I was six years old and my brother

Connie, aged four, died. It was a dark time in our home, and while he was sick and after he had died my mother lit a candle every evening in the centre of the big table in the parlour. A light of comfort and hope. It began a tradition in our family of: Let's light a candle. Over the years, my mother's children and grandchildren wrote to her from all over the world when they had a problem, asking her to light her candle. Even now when she is long gone, the practice continues and we light a candle in times of trouble.

So on the eve of this Palm Sunday I decide to light a candle in my front south-facing window onto the main road into West Cork, and another one in a side window looking onto the hill up to the church, a symbol of hope until this darkness is gone.

I continue to light it every evening just before the six o'clock news on RTE, which gives us the latest figures on the spread of corona and the number who have died in the previous twenty-four hours. While listening to the grim news I see the glowing candle and pray that this too will pass.

Our once-busy village, through which non-stop traffic usually flows, is now a quiet place, and as midnight approaches complete silence descends, except for an occasional car, delivery truck, ambulance, or Garda car. I look out at the now deserted village, which is as it was when I came here in1961. We have gone back in time. Before going to bed around midnight I put out the candles.

But then on Easter Saturday morning I get a sudden inspiration. Surely for Easter something bigger and more symbolic is desirable? Back up the corridor I have just the thing. Hoarders glow with justification when something buried in oblivion for years suddenly comes in useful. Now, maybe 'useful' is too strong a term, and probably 'find a use for' may be more correct, but either way I have just the thing to light up Easter in the cocoon.

It took twenty years of storage before this day of use has come about for my Big Boy. Back when the Millennium dawned, a giant candle which we christened Big Boy had been part of the Last Light Ceremony in our Parish Hall. We in Innishannon, like people all over the country, welcomed in the great new era of the new Millennium with a Last Light Ceremony. A candle to mark such a momentous occasion had to make a statement and this was how Big Boy came into my life. Standing on the floor he reaches to my hip and it takes the stretch of my two hands to encircle him, so he is indeed a Big Boy. He glowed for the Last Light

Ceremony and during the intervening years was regularly hauled out by male muscle for special candlelit occasions, of which we had many in our Parish Hall, St Mary's Church and Christ Church.

Now is the time to bring Big Boy forth again. But that's easier said than done because his cocoon in a room back the corridor is long, long way from the kitchen where a restoration is planned to prepare Big Boy for light-off. As you can gather, Big Boy is a serious weight, and my days of lifting big, heavy boys are long gone, so a plan has to be hatched. An able-bodied son could be asked to do the needful, but the same son regularly informs me that at some stage I am going to burn down the whole menagerie before calling it a day. So he's not an option, and in a cocoon options are limited.

I try a test lift and gasp in dismay, so lifting is definitely out. Dragging was the next option, so I catch Big Boy by the top of the head and pull him manually along the hallway, and when we eventually reach the kitchen it is possible to roll him along the floor to the table. But here is another challenge because lifting is unavoidable in getting Big Boy onto the table. Brain not brawn would have to come into play. First I tilt him sideways onto a chair, where he makes a rocky landing, and when he stops rocking I up-end him forwards onto the table, where he makes a crash landing. Alleluia! He is lying on his side on the table ready for surgery.

A pre-op inspection reveals that his wick is buried deep down in his gut in a rock-solid well of black wax. Internal surgery is required, so a hacking operation begins, of paring back layers of hardened candle grease to bring the wick to the level of its surroundings. A brutal job, in which knives of varied strengths, lengths and widths are tried and rejected. The operation takes over two hours amidst many regrets that this sorry state had been allowed to happen. But, eventually, after 'much blood, sweat and tears' and a bruised thumb joint, a level playing field is achieved, and to my surprise two wicks revealed! He has hidden twins. But two wicks is one too many and too smoky, so one will have to be eroded.

The next challenge is to get Big Boy to the front window, which is to be his glowing perch to welcome Easter. He is rolled off the table onto the chair and then he slides to the floor with a thump. On the floor there's plenty of space to roll, and eventually he is rolled to his destination. Too big for the window sill where for the past week the smaller candle has done a good job, Big Boy has to be tilted onto a small table inside the window.

On Easter Saturday night I light him and feel a glow of achievement. It is a very simple ceremony without the usual paschal fire outside the church, no incense, and no choir chanting the beautiful hymn 'The Light of Christ Has Come into the World'. No one but Big Boy and me.

Before going to bed that night I blow out the light of Big Boy and then have the bright idea that it might be easier to pare back his fresh wax build-up while he is warm and soft. But, on trying to ease him off his little table to get at it, Big Boy suddenly tilts sideways, sending out a waterfall of hot, scalding candle grease that just misses me. So I decide to postpone the pare-back operation until the following morning when conditions will be safer, though a lot more difficult. After a few more nightly tilts in the wrong direction, Big Boy is retired, and the original candle comes back into action. Sometimes smaller is better and definitely easier.

Easter Visitors

Late last summer before the corona genie got out of the bottle and the world was a different place, I got a phone call from a woman whom I had never seen or heard of, but she informed me that swifts were now an endangered species and that there was a need for something to be done about providing nest boxes for them in the village. Now, best to explain that if you are the 'elder lemon in the village' with your nose stuck in a lot of the goings-on that are none of your business, you may receive phone calls and emails about a large variety of subjects. Often these calls and emails come with attachments. One of my sons calls these jobs 'jumping monkeys' and advises passing them on as soon as possible. So I rang John, who lives up the hill behind me, and lectures on zoology in University College Cork. John is passionate about the care of our wildlife and since he came to live here has been a real boon to the village and to the bird life in the adjacent river valley and woods. I passed the buck on to John and then promptly forgot all about it. Never even asked over the following months what had happened about the swift boxes.

Now spring is here and I am well into cocooning, and watching out daily for the swirl of the swallows in my garden. Last year their arrival was vaguely noted, probably days after they had come, but this year I am looking forward to hearing the swish of their wings and watching their freedom of flight across the sky. Cocooning has sharpened our sense of appreciation of so many things that we previously took for granted or even completely ignored.

Then a phone call comes from John to say that the boxes for the endangered swifts had not got put up on the gable end of the Parish Hall as planned and now, due to corona, the hall was out of bounds. So a new plan is needed. A different location is required for the expected visitors who could arrive around Easter. John has their house already constructed and is looking for a site. Usually the procedure is, site first and then the building, but this is a ready-made house looking for a site. However, as with most new builds there were specifications attached, such as visibility from the road so that the swifts' arrival and progress could be easily monitored and noted by interested passersby. In corona country things that had previously gone unseen and unappreciated are now enriching lives.

Further up the hill from me and at the top of my garden is an old hall with its gable end facing onto the hill. Perfect, I think! But, as with most planning permissions, there is a problem with the location.

'Is there power in that old building?' John asks.

'No, but why would you want power?'

'We might need to plug in music to attract the swifts.'

Well! You learn something new every day! 'No power in there,' I tell him.

'What about the gable end of your house facing the hill, would you be okay with that?' John wonders.

'No problem,' I assure him, while privately wondering what the neighbours might think of the swifts' musical requirements.

'I can bring down the nesting box and show it to you later on. Will you be there this evening?'

'Where else would I be? I'm under house arrest,' I assure him. 'But I could be out in the garden, so shout in over the wall and I will go upstairs and put my head out the window to see your swift box and we can discuss proceedings.'

So that evening I am working in the garden and John

calls in over the wall. I go upstairs and put my head out the window at the furthest end of the house. As I do so a brainwave floats in: wouldn't balconies be a great addition to village houses? Corona was self-seeding improvisation of communication methods, so might it not be a good idea if future town developments were to incorporate balconies from which people could communicate and even hold mini-concerts and enter-tainments? Would I suggest this to Michael O'Flynn of O'Flynn Developments, a forward-thinking and imaginative man?

Down on the street John is standing, holding a narrow, oblong box with three front openings. It looks unobtrusive enough, but getting it up under the shoot is going to require a long ladder and a good sense of balance.

'Happy enough with that?' John asks.

'Looks grand, but what about their musical needs?'

'We'll get this box up first and then I'll figure that one out. I'll be back within a few days with a long ladder to put this up.'

'I'll be here,' I assure him.

That night I get the following email from John:

When to play Swift Calls CD/mp3

Swift calls can be played in the mornings and evenings on calm, dry days from May to July to good effect. However, as there are normally three waves of swift arrivals, these are the most effective times that I found to play the Swift Calls CD/mp3.

The first wave. These normally arrive in the last week in April–early May and consist mainly of breeding adults returning to their traditional nest sites. It is difficult to attract these to a new site (box) as they are extremely site faithful, however, displaced breeding adults will take up residency in new homes, but it's rare. You can play your CD/mp3 anytime from now but the chances of attracting any are slim.

The second wave. These start to arrive from the end of May and into the first half of June. These are the ones you are after. These are 2-3 year-old birds looking for a nest site. They are definitely attracted by the CD/mp3 calls and will fly up to investigate where the sound is coming from. Try and place your speakers as near as you can to your box and play it as loud as you can (with neighbours' agreement). Play whenever the weather is calm. Avoid wet and windy days as swifts don't prospect for new nest sites in bad weather. Best times to play your CD/mp3 is from 6 –11am and again from 8-10pm. If you're lucky enough to attract a pair they will spend the rest of the summer building a new nest ready for next year.

The third wave. These arrive in the middle of July. They are yearlings returning for the first time. They are interested in joining a colony and will visit several in the local area to suss out the best ones. They might even enter one of your boxes, roosting in it until they leave in August, but they won't start nest building until the following year. They are also attracted by the CD/mp3, so play as described above.

I read the above and it's comforting to know that we still have a few weeks in which to prepare for the particular swifts who have musical aspirations. In the meantime, it is all about getting the nest up so I wait to hear from John and comply with his plan. He's the expert.

It is now early April and each day is sunnier and more beautiful than the next. I am putting all my meals on a tray and eating out in the garden where it is a joy to sit and watch the birds in action. Having seats placed in different locations offers a variety of outdoor restaurants from which the garden and birds can be viewed. Though reared by a father who could name all the birds, I am a bit of an ignoramus in this context, so now is the time to change that. Up in the attic are books about birds that I poke out and bring into the garden to help me identify my entertainers. When you sit quietly in the garden without moving, the birds decide you're a garden ornament and totally ignore you. Despite my extreme ignorance, I do recognise some of them, but the migrants are beyond me, especially my little newcomer with the red hat. A blackbird is busy building in a clump of ivy on the wall of the old hall and another is perched on the roof of the shop next door. The guy on the roof is casting a wary eye around him, which seems a bit unnecessary at that height, and having assured himself that all is well he disappears in under a slate at the gable end. That pair have nested up there for years, and each year I watch to see the young emerge, but never see them take off, which leads me to think that young blackbirds take to the wing with no advance maternal flying lessons. But I might be wrong. A little wren is popping in and out of a hole between the stones on the wall of the old hall and I assume that they have a nest in there. They are high up and very safe from the neighbouring cats, who sometimes pay a visit. All the birds are singing as they build and fly around, and again I wonder why we no longer sing or whistle while we work, especially out in the open air. The birds, however, constantly sing and chirp as they soar and swish. It probably keeps them happy and it sure helps to keep us happy.

Then on Easter Saturday afternoon the swallows arrive. Sitting in the garden I suddenly hear the swish of wings. They are here! They soar high in the sky. My heart rises with them. They have arrived in time for the Resurrection. Alleluia!

That evening John rings to say that on Easter Monday evening he'll come with swift box, ladder and all the other necessary requirements. And hopefully a safe pair of hands, as yet unidentified, to hold the ladder. Gone are the days when I could rush out and offer to do the needful. Cocooners must stay in their cocoons! But I plug in a long lead in the room beside where the swifts will hopefully choose to reside. I am preparing to power their musical requirements.

But when John and his wife Amy, who is to be the ladder holder, arrive on Monday evening the long lead is needed for a more mundane job – to power the drill needed to erect the box. John very carefully climbs the extended ladder and marks the wall with precision, and then goes down again to bring up the drill. From the very top of the ladder John begins to press firmly on the drill and the ladder begins to vibrate off the wall. I hold my breath in case the ladder on which this wildlife expert, who was probably never meant to be double-jobbing as a steeplejack, might suddenly plunge earthwards. Then he looks across at me and asks very politely, 'Alice, can I have a glass of water, please?'

Oh holy Mother of God, I think. He's feeling dizzy and is about to topple off the ladder! So I run in sudden panic into the kitchen, find a glass, wash it furiously in case an old coronavirus might have landed on it, and then fill it with water and run to the window. I reach across to John with the glass, but in a very calm, polite voice he instructs: 'Put it on the window sill, Alice, where I can reach it, please.'

Which I do – and then he reaches the drill across and plunges the head into the water, remarking calmly, 'The bit was over-heating.' What a relief! And looking down at Amy I know that she had shared my anxiety.

Then the moment of truth is about to dawn when John mounts the ladder bearing the swift box. This is an additional balancing act, but is accomplished with remarkable composure. Then we three hold our breaths waiting to see if the box will slip effortlessly into the firmly erected holding brads. It does! We are ready for the swifts.

And hopefully their musical requirements will be in place too by the time the musically inclined ones arrive.

Beauty in the Eye
of the Beholder

The bluebells have arrived! For the past few days they have been creeping furtively into shady corners around the garden, gauging their reception, peeping out at me from behind sprouting ferns and dying daffodils, not quite sure of their welcome. Sizing me up and wondering how they will be received this year, remembering that last year they got a cool reception. Our relationship is not good because they are a bit like the children in the story *M'Asal Beag Dubh*, where the purchaser of a donkey agrees a fixed price plus a six-penny piece for every child in the encampment – and suddenly children appear from all corners! Bluebells too have the happy knack of being more numerous than originally anticipated. Their reputation for self-restraint is not good.

Now, *they* are woodland plants and *this* is a garden!

At least, that is my opinion, but the bluebells do not agree. And they may have a point. Because, originally, this was definitely a garden, but over the years, due to my lack of restraint in tree-planting, it may have changed into a woodland. This evolved without my realising it, but not so with the bluebells. They gleefully watched it happen and every year gained a little more ground. This, they were thinking, could be *our* place and all we have to do is persist, and she will eventually have to admit defeat. And they were right.

My cocooning is now their strength because my defences are down. Immediately on arrival they smell a change in the air. Cocooning has changed everything. Now there is more appreciation of little things, and simple things previously taken for granted or even unseen – or unwanted – are now absorbed and savoured.

The morning a few weeks ago when the beautiful white Bridal Wreath Spirea bush poured out over the stone wall by the garden gate I almost genuflected in awe at its beauty. Never before had it been so magnificent! Never before had its arrival met with such appreciation! Long, arching sprigs of flowers were reverently collected and arranged in a tall vase at the centre of the kitchen table and in the front hallway. It brightened and uplifted the cocoon. And I wondered how I would cope when Bridal Wreath would eventually depart, as depart she would, but there was no need to worry because on the first morning that she was about to say goodbye I walked further along the garden path and there in all her glory was the Pieris Forest Flame, bursting into brilliant bloom. Then further along was a mini Camilla with gorgeous white butterfly flowers swirling into bloom. I am ashamed to admit to not knowing the botanical name of this beautiful little bush, but nature carries on regardless of our ignorance. As all this was happening, the rest of the garden was unfolding and all the beautiful acers daily putting on their finery.

The acer is one of the most wonderful of garden trees, arriving before all the others, when the bleak days of winter are still chilling our bones. As these chilly days ease away, the acer begins to swirl soft lime-green clouds around her light, elegant limbs. And some acer limbs are rich red and amber, so even in their nude state they have a head-start, and it is a joy to watch them daily drape an additional layer over their beautiful branches.

Into all this abundance of nature crept the silent bluebells. And am I delighted to see them! My attitude has changed, changed utterly. Corona has put appreciative manners on me.

And so, after a few days of getting to know each other, and when they feel sure of their welcome, I am confident enough to take out a scissors and snip some of the long, delicate stems, gather a large bunch of them and ease them into an old glass jug on the kitchen table. Many years ago I found this lovely old jug with an imprint of ferns along its sides in an antique shop in Clonakilty, and it is the ideal recipient for garden flowers, especially when you feel somewhat apologetic about your previous lack of appreciation for the same flowers. Now I am saying *mea culpa*, so that the bluebells feel assured that this year they have come into a whole new world, into the realm of cocooning where they are very, very welcome indeed.

Feeling the need to share my delight in the vibrant arrival of the bluebells, I pick bunches of them and stand them into six tall, wide-necked bottles that were waiting to be recycled, and put them into a box, well spaced away from each other outside the front door. With them goes a sign stating that my garden is awash with bluebells, and inviting people to take a bunch, assuring them that the bottles have only been touched by well-washed hands. Just as I walk past my window I see a little girl outside with a happy smile on her face walking away with a bottle of bluebells. Thank heaven for little girls!

Cocooning Conversations

Cocooning has released reams of trapped conversations that have spent years imprisoned behind the bars of a frantic world too intent on stampeding to listen. Waves of unleashed words are flowing between friends who now have the gift of time because in the world of cocooning there is all the time in the world. Suddenly our speeding conveyor-belt life has crashed to a halt and we have been parachuted into silent cocoons with time on our hands. Hurry is locked out and we are locked in, with time to talk to each other and listen. All just a phone-call away. Now, when the phone rings, you sit down, put your feet up and enjoy the chat. Admittedly, the level of enjoyment has a lot to do with who is at the other end of the phone! This is certainly not the time for wet-day women.

A Cocoon with a View

Wet-day Woman

All her days were wet ones
And all her thoughts were sad,
And anytime you met her
You would regret you had.
She'd depress you drip by drip
And leave you feeling low,
Oh she is a wet-day woman
And will be always so.

Neither do you want to be conversing with a 'We'll all be ruined' prophet of doom. Or a bore whose interest in the world stops at himself. Oscar Wilde believed that the only unforgivable offence in life was to be boring. Never was that more true than in the world of cocooning. And as Oscar spent a long term in prison the world of cocooning was not entirely foreign to him.

In the early days of cocooning some of us may have been thinking short-term, but then Leo began to sound cautionary warnings and on 22 April informed us that 5 May, the anticipated date of release, might not now happen. I found myself humming, 'Those were the days, my friend, we thought they'd never end ...'.

And I am not sure if I was singing about the world of cocooning or the world before cocooning. Cocooning can lead to confused thinking.

One of the greatest gifts in life is a listening friend and how much more true is that in cocooning. Someone who is there when the world gets too much for us. And locked into cocooning, that world can regularly get too much for us. So when you fall into the 'poor me' zone and the phone rings, you pick it up cautiously, wondering who is at the other end – and breathe a sigh of relief when you hear a voice that is going to brighten up your cocoon. You find the nearest chair, collapse into it and soak up any crumbs of distraction that come your way.

In the early days of cocooning I had a conversation with my friend Phil, who remarked, 'It is resilience that will get us all through this' and, oh boys, have I often recalled her words. After many years of nursing and running a care centre for recovering alcoholics and drug addicts, she had 'looked at life from both sides now'. During cocooning, she and I have had many long conversations and I invariably come off the phone feeling better. She has mastered the art of positive living.

Having a 'Darina Allen' or 'Mary Berry' on call is a

great plus and the fact that she is a niece means that we can also discuss family matters. Eileen turns out super-duper brown bread and scones, an art I never mastered despite all my years in the kitchen. But a constant supply appears at my door. Her sister Treasa is the family archivist and we spend long hours in conversation on the phone digging up generations of long-gone Taylors and endeavouring to arrange them in historical sequence, a tall order once you go back beyond the horizons of a couple of centuries where one generation can easily get intermingled with another. So doing the family tree is a big challenge. Maybe the roots of many family trees could be planted and grown from our cocooning time?

Sean is another of my cocoon conversationalists. We go back a long way. When I came to live in Innishannon back in 1961, Sean and his little brother, Timmy, lived at the end of the village. Maybe because I was new and a bit at sea in my new surroundings, these two little lads semi-adopted me and we spent long hours together. They were great fun and full of the joys of life, and when my first-born arrived on the scene they took him out walking in his little stroller. Having left home well washed and looking pristine in blue baby outfits (as only a first-born can look), he invariable came back black as the hobs of hell, having had a great time visiting an old lady who was not into hygiene, where for hours he was literally as happy as a pig in muck.

In their teenage years Sean and Timmy worked during their summer holidays in our guest house. By then Sean had grown into a challenging teenager and he and I had constant battles of will. He was a kitchen devil and a dining room angel, who could charm the guests into slavish admiration of anything he put in front of them. In other words, he was designed for the catering business. Then he got a two-year scholarship to the Rockwell School of Catering, which was great. During this period he spent a summer season working as a trainee chef in a top-class hotel in Kerry and came home full of stories. One was about a young Kerry lad to whom one day the French chef was endeavouring to issue instructions in broken English about the refinements of his mashed potato requirements. The chef was failing to get his point across until a kindly Kerry woman working in the kitchen came to the young lad's rescue and translated: 'Pat, boyeen, he just wants you to make pandy.'

Later Sean opened up some top-class pubs and restaurants. During those years our lives ran on different tracks, but when my daughter thought that she might go into the catering business and was looking for holiday work experience, I rang Sean, who at the time had a pub and restaurant beside the GPO in Cork. She spent a happy summer working there and during that time Sean told her, 'The one thing that I learnt from your mother was that you can't recycle soap.' Apparently I must have felt that all the left-over little soap tablets from the bedrooms should not be dumped but recycled. I have a vague memory of shoals of small green soap tablets floating around in a large saucepan on the Aga, but no recollection of what happened to them after that. But from Sean's recollection it was not a success story.

Sean is great reader, with a wide interest in all that is going on in the world, he is good company and a great listener. The ideal cocoon conversationalist.

Another is priest friend, Denis, who is one of the inspirational priests who kept the flame of faith flickering while the Church self-destructed. His hope is that the world will go back to a new normal because the old normal was ruining the lives of young couples caught in a relentless spin of trying to balance the demands of high-pressure jobs with the needs of their young families.

In the cocoon, variety of subjects is the name of the game, and my lifelong friend Nora certainly provides that. Any time she rings I come off the phone either laughing, annoyed or raging, but never bored. She has an unorthodox opinion on a great variety of subjects above and beyond the range of my normal domain, and is convinced that we are all cramped by political correctness and live in an Ireland where no one is entitled to say what they think. She certainly does not fit into that category. A recent discussion with her was about the widespread practice of cheek-kissing that has crept into Irish society. Nora doesn't think much of it.

'Long ago the only ones who engaged in this cheek-pecking carry-on were maiden aunts, some of whom could not even stand the sight of each other,' she told me, 'and now we have these plastic-faced elderly statesmen from foreign countries, most of whom are bombing each other into extinction, and these guys then come on TV kissing each other. What the hell is all that about?'

'TV hosts do it all the time,' I told her. 'It seems be the acceptable thing to do now.'

'Well, it shouldn't be! We're like bloody sheep: one out the gate, all out the gate. Now it's even acceptable to jump into bed with someone who, a few hours earlier, was a total stranger. Sure that's pure bloody crazy. But can you open your mouth about it? No!' Nora was having a 'stop-the-world-I-want-to-get-off' day! Except that Nora did not want to get off until the world was in better shape than when she began the phone call.

A conversation with Annette is far less ruffling of the cocooning feathers because Annette thinks that we are all wonderful and that we are living at a great time. Even with corona on the rampage! She believes this too will pass and that in time all will be well again. And hopefully we may have learnt to love our world a little better. Annette is definitely a glass-half-full woman!

Cocooning conversations can give a varied view of the world outside. And now we have all the time in the world for them.

Then every few days there are family gatherings via Skype or Zoom onto which I am guided like a sleep-walker in the dark. But eventually I get there, and it is good to see the faces of family from faraway places. In some ways we have never been so interlinked as now. The miracle of modern communications is a great blessing in the cocoon.

Flowers of Freedom

Last Autumn when I was having one of my 'save the planet' days I went around the yard and garden and collected dried flower-heads off poppies, marigolds, sunflowers and many other nameless but well-loved varieties. Even went down on my knees to collect the nasturtium seeds that were scattered like confetti around the yard. Collecting nasturtium seeds is totally surplus to requirements as nasturtiums are so good at self-seeding that they are practically DIY seeds. They could almost come up through concrete, but because they were firm favourites of my mother's I have a soft spot for them. She probably loved them because gardening in the depths of North Cork prior to the arrival of garden centres was a case of the survival of the fittest, and nasturtiums certainly come into that category. But on that day in autumn last year my urge to propagate and collect the harvest was so strong that there was nothing in the garden safe from my foraging fingers. It is my yearly practice, but never before had I done it so extensively. And come this spring am I glad of that.

Sometimes spring can bring a special day when we feel in our bones that winter has finally decided to pack its bags and move on. The sun gets the message and comes out to warm and comfort us – and all of a sudden we are in the Garden of Eden. My mother called these 'pet days' and maybe that term came from the delicate baby animals that were especially loved and appreciated due to their early arrival and fragility, and so we often had pet calves and pet lambs. And now years later here in my Innishannon cocoon I have a pet day, for which I am so grateful.

Once the afternoon sun has come full south, it beams into my back yard and creates a sun pool. So I clear the wonky centre table of pots of departing daffodils, and give it a good clean down. This old table has seen many life changes since its creation by Uncle Jacky to be Aunty Peg's kitchen table. But it is still hanging in there and is now treated with the respect due to the frail and elderly. It certainly belongs in a cocoon. As does its other larger yard companion, now leaning against the shed that it needs to keep it standing. This old girl, which last year had its lower legs amputated due to foot rot, was evicted by my sister many years ago when she was converting her kitchen to minimalist living. This old lady too qualifies for cocooning.

Out of their neonatal chamber in the back porch I bring a diverse collection of seed containers and lay them out on Uncle Jacky's table. It seems right that his table is the platform for these little treasure-filled containers. He who created and fostered this garden, and whose apple tree that he planted as a young gardening enthusiast, will shortly be filling the garden with blossoms. His garden was a treasury of self-seeding. What blessings he left behind!

Now, with all the containers spread out like a future feast of flowers, I bring out a plump cushion from the kitchen couch and plonk it into a comfortable garden chair. This job is going to take time, and now I have all kinds of time.

The sun is warm on my back and I think of my late sister Ellen, who, whenever we were about to embark on an enjoyable experience, would rub her hands gleefully together and declare: 'Isn't this great.' So before getting going, I take time to savour my surroundings, the gorgeous red and yellow tulips glowing in the tubs around the yard. What a gift they are just now when my outdoor life is confined to this yard and garden. But how blessed am I to have this beautiful space. Never were gardens more appreciated than now. They are our chicken-runs. At night on TV I see people who are trying to cope in high-rise apartments and think what a ferocious challenge that is.

The roses are just beginning to leaf on the arch beside me. This arch was created with a black plastic pipe curved from the end of the garden shed to the corner of the back porch and supported by the legs of two retired Christmas trees. I learnt the 'art of making do' from Uncle Jacky because everything that came out of the garden he recycled back into the garden. Once a strong tree branch that he used to make a gate post sprouted and burst into leaf. My rose arch is not a thing of beauty but becomes invisible once shrouded with roses, and they are on their way. Nature is very forgiving of our human inadequacies, but I doubt that the trunks of my Christmas trees will ever spring into life.

The little acer in the central pot is beginning to unfurl its lovely, delicate leaves. The acer, being the first tree to emerge, brings comfort and hope when we are almost flattened by winter and so in need of a touch of spring. The hostas are beginning to peep up, but unfortunately the slugs are lying in wait. This year I am planning to new eradicator – Guinness. I had a spare bottle and filled a little tray with it, and the following morning found some drowned slugs. I know that sounds brutal, but it's either the slugs or the hostas, and drowning is supposed to be the pleasantest of exits. I sent out a request to the extended family to leave bottles or cans of Guinness at my door!

Some of the big flower pots have blank faces and often I have forgotten what they contain until they pop up their heads and say, 'Here I am.' Pots can be full of surprises, but unfortunately also full of weevil, and this year I am trying a new weevil exterminator – Jeyes Fluid. Uncle Jacky used it for a multitude of complaints, but this is my first year bringing it into action. It's the only weapon I can find in my back porch cupboard, which houses all kind of everything.

Once I start on my seed-sorting I realise that as well as the containers on the table I need extra receptacles to receive the contents of the various seed pods. A rummage through Aunty Peg's old corner press in the back porch unearths a collection of little wooden trays abandoned by an apprentice wood-turner as unfit for household display, but perfect now for the job on hand. It is a pure joy to watch the little waterfall of black poppy seeds pour from the dried pods into these little bowls. There is a multiplicity of seeds in each pod. One wonders how many of them will eventually spring into life, but even if only a tiny amount make it into flower how great would that be? The sunflower seeds are bigger boys and easier to handle, and the marigolds are a bundle of confusion and I'm unsure which are the pods and which are the seeds – so they all go in. The other anonymous ones are all kept separate and will later spring a surprise. I hope! But the nasturtiums are hardy lads and you can see how they survive as they overwinter with their coats on. They are ready for action. And so am I. The next step is planting.

Bhfuil cead agam dul amach?

In cocooning you have to be very selective about what you tune into on radio and TV because an overdose of the wrong mix could pitch you into the twilight zone. We are very vulnerable in cocooning, and preserving the equilibrium is hugely important because you cannot afford to succumb to the 'poor me' scenario, as there is no cure mechanism in the cocoon, only yourself. Needless to mention, the same applies to newspapers, that is if you are one of those antiques, like me, who still reads them. Turning myself into a well-informed financial wizard by reading the business columns will not ease the financial stresses of the world only succeed in giving me high blood pressure. And now there is no way of getting out for the cure of retail therapy or a walk in the woods!

Listening to a good radio programme can give you

a mental lift and by being careful you can cherry-pick what best suits you. But despite this advice to myself, last night I watched a programme on the life of a brilliant broadcaster who had simply burnt out. I had not expected this programme to be so disturbing and went to bed not entirely at ease with myself, and was awakened in the small hours by a disturbing nightmare, and when I finally got back to sleep it was only to find myself outside a jail watching a fresh-faced young man going in, and wondering what it would do to him.

So before pressing a button or turning knobs on entertainment or information, caution is the name of the game. Six weeks of cocooning makes one fragile. Sunday morning on RTE radio is usually upbeat, and last Sunday morning it was wonderful to listen to Mícheál Ó Muircheartaigh read Brendan Kennelly's poem 'Begin Again'. I have always loved that poem and in today's situation it is so relevant. We are all wondering right now when we can begin again! In school long ago when we needed to go out to the toilet we shot up our hand with the request: '*Bhfuil cead agam dul amach?*' Now we are all waving our hands at Tony Holohan and pleading: '*Bhfuil cead agam dul amach?*'

On the same station last Sunday morning John Bowman was celebrating fifty years of Listowel

Writers' Week, and I found hearing the voices of Brian McMahon and John B. Keane very uplifting. It was a programme full of wisdom and humour.

The 6pm News is almost compulsive listening to keep abreast of developments in corona country. I feel slightly uneasy and queasy while waiting for the latest corona figures from the Health Board. I'm not quite sure how to explain this uneasiness but there is a touch of the 'Romans watching the Christians being thrown to the lions in the Colosseum' about it, or an element of reminiscence of that time in history when people went to watch hangings. It is slightly unnerving to sit there waiting to hear of the numbers who have died, and the new cases diagnosed. These public death lists are transfixing and horrifying.

I am slightly relieved when the news is over and the weather forecast comes on, as this focuses the mind forward to tomorrow. Then it is possible to do a quick survey across all channels to see what might be available that could keep one positive, informed and entertained. While in the cocoon, 'Nationwide' is always uplifting viewing, as is 'Ear to the Ground', and 'Home of the Year' satisfies my nosey desire to get a peep in behind other people's front doors, as does the old house restorations.

A Cocoon with a View

Now that I am deprived of visits to craft and antique shops, I have become addicted to 'Salvage Hunters' and as Drew Pritchard traverses the country searching for antique finds I am a backseat passenger. Going along with him and his co-host to visit the great homes and antique shops of England is highly entertaining. I always harboured a secret desire to run an antique shop, and with 'Salvage Hunters' I share Drew's unquenchable thirst for rare and wonderful objects, and am delighted when he discovers a gem. A weekly dose of Monty Don is a must, and I love the Friday-night ramble around Long Meadow. Then out of the blue a friend sent me a link to an hour and a half in Monet's garden. Oh joy of joys, I thought I was in heaven. And the beauty of this heaven is that I can make return visits. Manna in the cocoon!

'Portrait Artist of the Year' on Sky Arts is a constant source of delight, and the amazing miracles that these artists create on canvas are illuminating, while at the same time reminding me of the canvas and paints upstairs waiting for me to make an enjoyable mess. On Sky Arts one can come across some wonderful performances to transport you out of the cocoon for hours. One night I happened across an amazing performance of 'The Phantom of the Opera' and after the show all the previous Phantoms, including our own Colm Wilkinson, came on stage and gave spine-tingling performances, accompanied by the golden-voiced leading ladies in magnificent costumes, and then Andrew Lloyd Webber himself joined them. It was a rare feast of delights. Every week I have a fix of 'Mastermind', and am mesmerised by the black chair, even though the chances of being able to answer even one question asked by John Humphrys would be a bit of a miracle. And, of course, on all stations wildlife programmes build extensions onto the cocoon.

Recently on the BBC they have taken to quoting the poem 'Don't Quit', which is an old favourite of mine. I was a bit surprised to hear this on the BBC who, I thought, might have considered themselves a bit too suave for such simplicity, but then Covid-19 has changed everything. This poem urges us to stick in there when life is at its toughest and to simply keep on doggedly keeping on, especially when you feel like throwing in the sponge and lying down in a pool of despair. Because right around the corner, from our darkest hour, the sun is beginning to rise. And life will get good again. So don't give up now, but keep crawling forward and you will get there. If you give up now you will never reach that sunny place waiting for you right around the corner where life will be good again. So Don't Quit!

How am I doing? How are we all doing? That is the question!

In pre-corona days, which now seem like a century ago, that query was more a vague salutation than a question. But no more! Now it is a genuine enquiry. As if we have all suddenly been shot into a strange new world having acquired a rare precarious condition requiring constant mental health checks. Which is indeed true. Back in normal times the reply to that question was sometimes: 'As good as can be expected.' Nobody gives that answer now, simply because nothing about this world was expected and we have no idea how we are expected to be.

As in *Alice in Wonderland*, we seem have somersaulted down a brown burrow into a weird new world. But, unfortunately, down here there is no white rabbit, only an invisible monster stalking around trying to kill as many of us as he can get at. The only solution was to lock ourselves in and at first that direction only applied to the fragile and elderly (like me), and when this proved insufficient as the spiky monster was still able to get his tentacles in many open doors, everyone was then asked to stay at home and lock him out.

At first we complied and all banded together in a great wave of togetherness to mind the most vulnerable and to support our amazing health-care workers, who are on the front line of defence, but now maybe we are beginning to get a bit complacent, and as the weather is beautiful we are getting restless. There is a new scientific system by which human activity on the earth's surface can be ascertained, and it shows that there are too many of us out and about. But I can see that for myself from the traffic increase last weekend on the road outside my window. Simon Harris and Tony Holohan are pleading desperately with us all to stay at home and stop this monster killing more of us. Will we comply or will cabin fever drive us all to do crazy things? Have we too many Mad Hatters?

As I write this I suddenly hear horses' hooves on the street outside my widow. I listen carefully in case I am finally losing it, but, no, that is unmistakably the sound of stamping hooves. As I rise from my chair to check out this strange scenario, a horse's rump appears against the window pane and then a second horse's head comes into view. A young girl is holding them, and I assume that another person has gone into the shop next door. The horses are perfectly at ease in this new traffic-free zone, and I see a local farmer mounting a tractor after a leisurely ramble across the road with his messages. Not a car in sight! We have definitely gone back in time.

Then comes a knock on my window and a neighbour's smiling face appears, and she points to my door. When I open it cautiously and peep out, she has moved on and outside is a bag of scones and a pot of jam, with a cheery message on a homemade card. Also included is a little packet of honesty seeds from her garden. Thank heaven for good neighbours.

A Swift Flew over the Cuckoo's Nest

This morning on stumbling into the bathroom I glance sideways at the mirror and a strange sight looks back out at me. A bleary-eyed mess with a shaggy grey mane hanging like a line of wet washing along the shoulders is not a pleasant sight to behold first thing in the morning. Not a vision to uphold the self-esteem. A bad hair day. Definitely going to seed! You could go cuckoo in a cocoon if you lose the grip. Something just has to be done. Done right away. As I am a creature of impulse, immediate action is taken. The only scissors available, other than useless nail scissors, are my gardening scissors that substitute as a pruner when my roof garden needs a stop put to its gallop. Originally hefty dress-making scissors, they have gone through many reincarnations before finally finishing up as a gardening accessory. So I bring them in from their customary location in my weed-collecting bucket on the roof and return to the viewing mirror. Then I take a good look at the cutting possibility of the scissors – and discover, to my horror, that they are filthy. Probably laden with bugs too! Could one of them be corona? I give them a fast scalding under the hot tap while wishing myself happy birthday.

Then I study the wild-meadow woman in the mirror, take a deep breath and begin to mow around the headlands. First tentatively along the dangling growth under the right ear, being careful to avoid the ear, and then progress steadily around the back bend. There the scissors disappear from view, going into invisible territory along the base of the pole, where they have to be guided by neck contours. Then, gaining confidence and momentum, they gather speed. Swathes of grey begin to cascade onto the floor. Then around to left-ear territory, and steering around to the back with instinct as the guide. The fall-out is alarming as widespread showers of grey snow float to the bathroom floor. Have to keep going now, cannot chicken out with a half-shorn head. Eventually all the headlands around the head are mown. And how does the head in the mirror look? Almost afraid to look. But then, slowly, chance a cautionary glance. Not half bad!

Then for the big one! The fringe. This is make-or-break territory. My frontal fringe from beneath which I have struggled for a clear view of the world in recent days, has to be shortened by a good inch or two. Definitely need to clear that window onto the world. I stoop forward over the washbasin and my fringe swings out over my eyes like a grimy net curtain. This is definitely cutting in the dark territory, but the scissors plough through the fringe, like an old-fashioned farmer's scythe through a hedge of nettles. A further shower of grey snow pours into the washbasin. Then a return journey to trim and straighten the edges. Finished! I'm almost afraid now to raise my head to view the result, but eventually take a deep breath, raise my eyes with apprehension to see the woman in the mirror. My mother's face is looking back out at me. I am delighted to see her. It's such a pleasant surprise to see her in the mirror, I feel like singing: 'My mama told me there'd be days like this'. My father had done the needful in her hair world and when her daughters could wield the scissors we took over the job. Good skin and hair were in her genes, but beautifying herself was not high on her list of priorities, so honey and cider vinegar took care of her beauty requirements.

A Cocoon with a View

Made brave by my success so far, I decide on a general overhaul of the body – a repairs and maintenance job. Very important while cocooning. Looking good often means feeling good. So nails – hands and toes – are next in line and then a general overhaul job in all departments needing attention. Then into the shower where clinging bits of grey are douched away in a lather of soap and shampoo. Boys! But that feels good! Then for the final flow, when I slowly turn the shower towards cold, and then colder, bracing myself for the final twist of the shower knob when a truly cold sheet of water hits my head and a freezing spray of sleet belts unmercifully down on me. Wow! I stick it for as long as I can and then, with a gasp of relief, step out of the shower and gratefully grasp the big bath towel. It feels good to be alive. The shorn hair blow-dries to a smooth white thatch. A bit like Friar Tuck of yesteryear! Ready for another day in the cocoon.

Later I get an email from John, the swift-music man, telling me that it is time to install their sound system. A vague time later in the day is arranged and just before six a shout comes over the garden wall. I head up the stairs to open the window of what I now think of as the swift room. Down below in the street is John, with leads and little boxes dangling across his shoulders. After a pleasant window-to-street conversation catching up with various village activities, we decide on a plan of action to get all the gear that John has below up to me at the window. Unlike Rapunzel, especially after this morning's shearing, I cannot reach down my hair, so a plan of action comes into play. My first thought is a basket, but decide that a basket could have a mid-air wobble and that a deep bag would be a safer option. So I retrieve a light, deep bag (glad to be a hoarder!) and tie the two handles with a long, light rope (glad to be a hoarder again!) and ease the bag down to John. He then gives instructions from the ground up on how procedures are to be carried out when his valuable cargo arrives up to me. At this point it has to be admitted that I am not an apt mechanical student and even more so in the world of electronics. But John does not know that, and I did not have the heart to tell him. Sometimes ignorance is bliss and John was on a swift run (pardon the pun) and I did not want to dampen his enthusiasm. Maybe he might never find out that he is dealing with a woman off Noah's Ark! I fish up the bag of electronic tricks and land it carefully on a nearby table. I begin to carry out John's highly specific instructions as he shouts them up from the street below. Then, as I follow his extremely clear guidelines, I begin to appreciate that John has spent many years enlightening ignoramuses like me, and has mastered his skills perfectly. So all is accomplished in jig-time, but to John's consternation no sound is forth-coming from our swift music system. He is perplexed, but to be honest I am not in the least bit surprised, simply because I am always truly amazed when these things work anyway! On John's instructions, I send the cargo back down again to be rechecked by him, and in the easing down process mindlessly (yes, I know that I'm practising mindfulness) let go of my fishing-rod rope, so now there is no way of hauling it back up again. But John is nothing if not resourceful and, having rechecked his swift sound system, he winds the rope into a tight ball and shoots it up to me in the open goal. But I am no Packie Bonner, so I miss the ball, which bounces back down to John. But better luck the next time and I haul in the loot, unpack the bag and replug everything. Suddenly the Angelus bell in the church up the hill begins to peal – and John lis-tens attentively. The apparatus has been timed to go on at six o'clock as a trial run, so now the time is right – and then it begins to chirp like a happy bird. Amazing!

John had jokingly promised Mozart, and that it definitely is not, neither is it Pavarotti or the 'Fields of Athenry'. But hopefully the neighbours will like it, and its chirping melody will catch the ear of the swooping swifts. We await their arrival.

Sanity-savers in the Cocoon

Everybody needs a rage buddy. Especially now. This morning I need one so badly. But right now you can't go venting your frustration on others because in this coronavirus realm that is a luxury in which we cannot indulge, because everyone else is doing their best to keep afloat in the same troubled waters. But a fever is in my mind and it's not corona fever – or at least I hope not – but with cabin fever you can convince yourself that you have a multitude of fevers. I thought of my old friend's approach: stand back calmly and ask 'What's to be done?' But I want to do nothing, only wallow in my misery. Then I remember my mother's positive comment whenever we tackled a challenging job; she would declare 'Isn't it great that we have the mind on us to do it.'

This morning I have the mind on me to do precisely nothing. Cabin fever has sneaked in under the door and is lapping around my mind. I cannot indulge myself in complaining as I feel that there are so many other people in more difficult situations than mine. But, as our beloved village doctor, Dr Cormac, used to quote, '*Níl aon tóin tinn mar do thóin tinn féin*' which translated means 'There's no sore arse like your own sore arse.' And this morning mine is very sore! I need a sanity-saving project because otherwise I am going to murder someone, and in a cocoon there is no one to murder only yourself. Wafting around aimlessly in a cocoon is a recipe for disaster, so a sanity-saving strategy is vital. But how to get started? I need the prod of something that is really annoying me to get me going.

So do a survey of my surroundings trying to ascertain what is annoying the hell out of me and what do I really need to get done? Then it strikes me like a bolt from the blue: the windows! I hate dirty windows and always want to be able to see the world outside through sparkling glass. How much more important is that now when a clear view of the outside world is vital for our state of mind? The windows at the back of the house overlooking the yard and garden frame the pleasures outside as you walk by them. Now they are clouded with winter grime. They are crying out to be cleaned. But can I motivate myself to begin? Not this morning! But could Brendan Kennelly be right: is there in us all an irrepressible urge to begin again? This is testing time! So, with more dogged determination than motivation, a window-cleaning session is begun. At first tentatively and slowly, but gradually my engine begins to warm up, and as one window after another begins to clear so does my state on mind. As I travel along from one window to the next, the pictures hanging on the walls between the windows get a swipe of a cleaning cloth *en route*. With all the windows done, my engine is beginning to purr, so I decide to tackle the silver on the table at the end of the hall. Then I feel that while I am doing that, the dishwasher could be simultaneously doing another job. So I load that up with a collection of dusty ware off the top of the old chest in the corner of the hall.

I then collect all the pieces of silver and lay them out on top of the newspaper-covered kitchen table. Usually, cleaning the silver is a job to be done as quickly as possible. But not today. Today is different. I am going to take my time and savour the actual doing. This assortment of bits and pieces is the collection of a lifetime. Each has its own story, and as I polish I am going to listen to their stories. The biggest and most elegant piece is very difficult to describe, but the two words that come to mind are 'ornamental' and 'useless'. It has a tall, tulip-shaped centre, with smaller branches arching outwards from a circular base, and, apart from looking magnificent, has no practical use that one could possibly imagine. It was acquired by a practical sister in a moment of sheer madness at an auction, but after a few years of questioning her sanity on that particular day and refusing to maintain it in the regal state which it demanded, decided to off-load it. So I was informed that it was to be mine because I was the only member of the family to be leisurely enough and crazy enough to be still polishing silver. It sits in regal state at the end of my hallway and I love its beautiful uselessness. After all, not everything in life has to be functional and productive. Now it is polished until it shines brighter than it has ever shone before, and in the process it is thanked for all the visual pleasure that it has given me over the years. Next, a little silver frame, falling apart but trying valiantly to hold within its fragile contours a photo of my mother sitting in the sun in her garden. I remember buying this frame at an antique fair and paying far too much for it, but there was something about its quirkiness that appealed to me. My mother, who was of a practical turn of mind, would have been horrified that her picture-frame cost so much! Then comes an unrecognisable young me with our eldest on his First Holy Communion Day. I peer at my unrecognisable face and decide that back then I had a very unlived-in face that looked as if it had a lot to learn about life. Not sure if I learned it though! But it's a lovely frame! On to the next piece, which is a little silver plate purchased in Egan's of Cork in 1972 to celebrate the fortieth wedding anniversary of Uncle Jacky and Aunty Peg. This brought back happy memories of a family gathering on 23 April of that year. All the children were young, and the celebrating couple fit and well. It was a great day and turned out to be our last happy occasion together, because within a few years Jacky and Peg had both died. An ordinary day which, in retrospect, was far from ordinary. This plate, engraved to commemorate it, is now a happy memory of them. Another plate was presented to me by the English Class of St Brogan's College, Bandon, with whom I did a reading back in 1988. That was a very special day, as they were a super group of Honours English students with an amazing teacher, Eileen Corkery, who went on afterwards to be an inspirational headmistress. Then, in a modern Newbridge frame that practically self-polishes, is a photo of Ellie and myself in peals of laughter on a family outing to Parknasilla a few years ago.

When all are satisfactorily gleaming, back they go onto the top of the old credenza where they sparkle in the reflecting mirror behind them. By then the dishwasher is done and the glowing ware can be returned to the top of the old chest. The sun shines in through the sparkling windows – and I am no longer in need of a Rage Buddy. The sanity-saver has worked, and Brendan Kennelly has been proved right.

May Day in the Cocoon

It is the first day of May. I have always loved May Day as it holds the key to summer in its flowery pocket. However, this May Day is going to be very different, though the bluebells are still vibrant and the trees are flouncing into swirling fresh layers.

Today brings back memories of other May Days. To May Days of childhood when we were allowed, at last, to take off our long stockings and heavy boots and go barefoot to school through the fields for the first time. Oh the delight of that freedom. Up to that date, no matter how warm the weather, my mother held fast and forbade us to 'cast a clout'. But come the first of May, the long-awaited day was here and we were free. Free to dance through wet grass. To feel the warm dew run down our legs and in between our toes. There is no delight equal to dancing barefoot through warm grass that connects us with the sacredness of the earth through our bare feet. On that day the young calves were also set free from the confines of their now smelly straw house. At first they were dazzled by day-light and stood mesmerised on the threshold, and then, suddenly, they realised that there was another world out there beyond the restricting confines of this straw-filled world. They shot out the door, hoisting their rumps skywards and cocking their tails in the air, to run in sheer exultation down the new-found fields of freedom and dance around in circles of free abandon-ment. We and the calves were at one in our apprecia-tion of May Day.

But we children had the added excitement of making a May altar, which filled us with anticipation, so we rushed home from school to get started. Our enthusiasm may not have been entirely motivated by religious fervour, nevertheless it resulted in a statue of Our Lady being raised high on a large box draped with one of our mother's best tablecloths and surrounded by jampots overflowing with bluebells and buttercups.

On the days leading up to May Day in the cocoon, I knew that running barefoot through early-morning grass was not an option as the squad car now sta-tioned at the end of the village checking movements might put a stop to my bid for freedom. But cocooning had unearthed another emotional memory as well, the desire to create a May altar. I had not made one since childhood, but cocooning had stimulated a seed of remembrance and that idea began to blossom. It brought back memories of Frank Patterson singing the hymn 'Bring Flowers of the Fairest' which Gay Byrne always played on his morning show on May Day.

Bring flowers of the rarest,
Bring blossoms the fairest,
From garden and woodland
And hillside and dale;
Our full hearts are swelling,
Our glad voices telling
The praise of the loveliest
Flower of the vale.

O Mary! we crown thee with blossoms today,
Queen of the angels, Queen of the May.
O Mary! we crown thee with blossoms today
Queen of the angels, Queen of the May.

That song invariably brings back memories of May processions and little girls adorned in their First Holy

Communion dresses, delighted to be parading around looking angelic.

I am not sure what format a May altar may take in my cocoon but feel that as the day progresses an altar plan will unfurl in my mind.

In the meantime the roof garden needs to be planted as May Day is here, and the sooner the seeds are in the better. But when I go outside on the roof to assess the work involved I am horrified to see a cat stalking along the top of another roof across the yard, at the end of which a blackbird has a nest full of baby chicks under the slates. The blackbird is now cackling in alarm at the sight of the cat who is striding balefully in her direction. A loud yell in the cat's direction temporarily halts his stride and he stops short to look across at me and ascertain how much of a threat I am to his planned attack. He knows immediately that at this distance I am pretty ineffective, so instant and more powerful intervention is demanded to stop him in his killing tracks. I quickly whip off my shoe and shoot it, spiralling in his direction, which sends him tumbling down the side of the roof onto the ground and high-tailing it up into the garden. The blackbird is safe.

While recovering from the cat attack I collapse into a chair on my roof and wait for the blackbird to reappear, just to reassure myself that all is well. Within minutes she is back on the roof opposite with a beak full of wriggling worms, so all is definitely well in her world. Then I retrieve my shoe from the yard down below, collect my seed trays, and proceed with my planting in the boxes and pots on the roof. No fresh compost in this year of making-do with what we have – even Monty Don, who is a big advocate of fresh replacement, has advised on yielding to the limitations of cocooning. Planting requires a lot of kneeling and rising, and makes me aware that my hinges are getting rusty, and, as one of my sons constantly reminds me, I am no spring chicken. So, when all is accomplished, I am grateful to sit in the sun and admire my roof-top view, which at the moment includes the scaffold-ing-enwrapped top of The Woodview pub next door that is having a reincarnation, which at the moment has come to a halt due to Covid-19 restrictions. This affords the enterprising crows an opportunity to take advantage of the temporary respite and they are busy erecting a housing estate in the chimneys. I would like to convey to them that all their efforts might be in vain as they could be evicted before moving-in date. All depends on the unfolding of restrictions.

Beyond the bandaged head of the The Woodview,

the elegant steeple of Christ Church peers through the trees and then all is woodland, for which I am extremely grateful to the former owner of The Spires who planted extensively, and then we were extremely lucky that the developer left the trees untouched and built around them, so now, instead of viewing rows of houses, we have a rich woodland view and the home owners are surrounded by mature trees. We sometimes need to be very grateful for the foresight of those who came before us.

Recovery time over, preventive steps now need to be taken to stop my friend the blackbird from uprooting all the seeds in the early hours while I am still in the land of nod. A poke around in the garden shed unearths rolls of green plastic wire, used years previously to deter my dogs Kate and Lolly from the same practice. But the coverings for these rooftop containers need to be much smaller, so the wire has to be cut into the required lengths. The big scissors, that a few days earlier had done the needful with my hair, again come out of the bucket and they run effortlessly through the pliable plastic wire. With this job done and all the seeds safe from my friend the blackbird, my thoughts turn back to the May altar.

While seed-planting, a plan had come into my

head when my eye fell on a large statue of the Blessed
Virgin resting on a shelf beside the exit door to the
roof. Instead of bringing the flowers from the garden
in to decorate the May altar, why not take Mary out
to the flowers? This is no little Mary, but a tall, sub-
stantial lady with an interesting story! She was won by
Aunty Peg and Uncle Jacky in a raffle, which sounds
a bit unbelievable in today's Ireland. The raffle took
place prior to 1961, because she was here before me,
and was much loved by Jacky and Peg. Because of
her story, I have a soft spot for her, and had recently
wondered about her chances of survival subsequent to
my demise. So maybe a decision today might secure
her future and provide an opportunity for her to live
out her days in Uncle Jacky and Aunty Peg's garden.
With this decision made, I reach up and lift her down
from her perch. She's heavier than anticipated, so we
stagger along the corridor together and come very
slowly downstairs. A missed step or wobble and we
could have a crash-landing. Grateful to be cocooning,
because there will be no unexpected caller to question
my movements or my sanity.

Mary and I make it slowly to the garden gate, taking
occasional breaks along the way so that I can draw
my breath and regain my balance and equilibrium,

until eventually we stand together at the gate and view the garden. The next step is choice of location! This choice has to be right the first time round as this is no time to go waltzing around the garden because Mary and I could well come a cropper on the rough stone paths and steps! And I am a ditherer! It takes me a long time to make up my mind, but this is a luxury to be ruled out in the present circumstances. So I do a mental survey of potential sites. St Joseph, already in location, is a very classy Joseph made of Portland stone, and even though my Mary is big, he is bigger still, and now beautifully weathered in the outdoors, whereas Mary has the pale look of someone confined too long indoors. All the other occupants of the garden have mellowed into their surroundings, whereas Mary will stand out like Hamlet's ghost. So the choice of location needs to be a shadowy bower to blend her into this new outdoor world.

Leaving Mary standing at the gate I do a garden walkabout, and different sites are selected and then eliminated. Site-hunting for an ordinary mortal is one thing, but searching for a home to accommodate someone accustomed to heavenly realms is a challenging task. Eventually a decision is reached and a shaded location beneath a tree, with her back to the stone wall of the old Methodist hall, is the choice. Mary and I stagger to the chosen spot, where a level foundation is scooped out, and a few flat stones placed beneath her toes effect a secure balance. Supported by the Methodist wall, with Joseph within calling distance, and surrounded by bluebells, it's the perfect location. But like Covid-19 that could change in the days ahead.

That evening, while Mary was still finding her feet in the garden, Leo appeared on the steps of Leinster House to tell us that the outdoor human run was being extended and that the likes of me could emerge out of lockdown on 5 May!

Might we cocooners, like the calves, be at first dazzled by daylight, then kick our heels in the air, make a leap of exuberance and take off in a flight for freedom across the fields?

The great escape!